DR. STEVEN J. MIDDLETON

Gut Health With A Plant Based Diet

The Comprehensive Plant-Based Guide to Reducing Bloating, Improving Digestion, and Living Your Best Life

This book was professionally typeset on Reedsy.
Find out more at reedsy.com

Contents

About the Author

Dr. Steven J. Middleton is a highly accomplished and respected doctor specialized in gastroenterology and nutrition. With a passion for promoting optimal gut health, Dr. Armando has dedicated his career to helping individuals improve their well-being through a plant-based approach.

As an advocate for holistic health, Dr. Middleton believes in the power of lifestyle interventions, particularly the role of nutrition in promoting overall well-being. His approach combines evidence-based medicine with a deep understanding of the body's intricate systems, allowing him to provide personalized and effective recommendations for his patients.

Introduction

Dear Reader,

Welcome to the transformative world of gut health and plant-based living! I am thrilled to embark on this journey with you as we explore the incredible power of nourishing our bodies with a plant-based diet. In this comprehensive guide, we will delve into the fascinating realm of gut health, unraveling the secrets to reducing bloating, improving digestion, and ultimately, living your best life.

Now, you might be wondering, why should I care about my gut health? Well, let me share a personal story that ignited my passion for this topic. A few years ago, I found myself constantly battling digestive issues - the uncomfortable bloating, the unpredictable bouts of indigestion, and the nagging feeling that something just wasn't right. It was frustrating, to say the least, and it took a toll on my overall well-being.

But then, I discovered the remarkable connection between gut health and a plant-based diet. It was like stumbling upon a hidden treasure trove of wellness. As I began to incorporate more plant-based foods into my daily meals, I noticed a profound shift in my digestive health. The bloating diminished, my digestion became smoother, and I felt an incredible surge of energy and vitality. It was a revelation.

This personal experience sparked a deep curiosity within me, leading me to dive headfirst into the world of gut health research. I devoured scientific studies, consulted with experts, and experimented with various plant-based recipes. And now, armed with knowledge and personal experience, I am here to guide you on your own journey towards optimal gut health.

In this book, we will not only explore the fundamentals of gut health but also uncover the transformative power of a plant-based diet. Together, we will navigate the intricacies of the digestive system, understand the role of gut microbiota, and discover the incredible array of plant-based foods that can heal and nourish our bodies from within.

But this book is not just about theory and scientific jargon. It is about making gut health accessible and achievable for everyone, regardless of their background or dietary preferences. Whether you are a seasoned plant-based enthusiast or new to the concept, this guide is designed to be your trusted companion, providing practical tips, delicious recipes, and evidence-based insights that will empower you to take charge of your gut health.

So, get ready to embark on a journey that will not only transform your digestive health but also enhance your overall well-being. Say goodbye to bloating, discomfort, and digestive woes, and say hello to a vibrant, energized, and thriving you.

Are you ready to unlock the secrets of gut health and embrace a plant-based lifestyle? Let's dive in together and discover the incredible potential that lies within each and every one of us.

<u>Why Gut Health Matters</u>

When it comes to our overall well-being, we often focus on factors like diet, exercise, and mental health. But there is one crucial aspect that is often overlooked, yet holds the key to our vitality and vitality: gut health. Yes, you heard it right - your gut health is more than just a matter of digestion. It is a complex ecosystem that plays a pivotal role in your physical and mental well-being.

So, why is gut health important? Let's delve into the fascinating world of your gut and uncover the reasons why nurturing it should be a top priority.

1. Digestion and Nutrient Absorption: Your gut is responsible for breaking down the food you consume, extracting essential nutrients, and absorbing them into your bloodstream. When your gut is healthy, it efficiently carries out these processes, ensuring that your body receives the vital nutrients it needs to function optimally. On the other hand, an unhealthy gut can lead to digestive issues like bloating, gas, constipation, or diarrhea, hindering the absorption of nutrients and leaving you feeling sluggish and depleted.

2. Immune System Support: Did you know that approximately 70% of your immune system resides in your gut? Your gut acts as a barrier, protecting your body from harmful pathogens and toxins. A healthy gut microbiota, the community of microorganisms living in your gut, helps maintain a robust immune system, preventing infections and diseases. Conversely, an

imbalance in gut bacteria can weaken your immune response, making you more susceptible to illnesses.

3. Mental Health and Mood Regulation: Have you ever experienced a "gut feeling" or noticed how your emotions can impact your digestion? Well, there's a reason for that. Your gut and brain are intricately connected through the gut-brain axis, a complex communication network. The gut produces neurotransmitters like serotonin, often referred to as the "happy hormone," which plays a crucial role in regulating mood and emotions. A healthy gut contributes to balanced neurotransmitter production, promoting mental well-being and reducing the risk of conditions like anxiety and depression.

4. Inflammation and Chronic Disease: Chronic inflammation is at the root of many diseases, including autoimmune disorders, cardiovascular conditions, and even certain types of cancer. An unhealthy gut can trigger chronic inflammation, as imbalances in gut bacteria can lead to increased permeability of the intestinal lining, allowing toxins and bacteria to enter the bloodstream. This can set off an inflammatory response throughout the body, contributing to the development of chronic diseases.

5. Weight Management and Metabolism: Maintaining a healthy weight is not just about calories in versus calories out. Your gut health influences your metabolism, appetite regulation, and even the storage of fat. Studies have shown that an imbalance in gut bacteria can lead to weight gain and obesity. On the other hand, a healthy gut microbiota can support weight management by promoting a healthy metabolism and reducing cravings for

unhealthy foods.

These are just a few of the many reasons why gut health is crucial for your overall well-being.

The Transformative Power of Plant-Based Nutrition

A plant-based diet, rich in whole, unprocessed plant foods, can be a game-changer when it comes to nurturing your gut health. By shifting your focus towards plant-based nutrition, you provide your gut with the essential tools it needs to thrive. Let's explore how a plant-based diet can support and improve your gut health:

1. Abundance of Fiber: Plant foods are naturally abundant in dietary fiber, which is essential for a healthy gut. Fiber acts as a prebiotic, providing nourishment to the beneficial bacteria in your gut. This promotes the growth of a diverse and balanced gut microbiota, which is crucial for optimal digestion and overall well-being. By consuming a variety of fruits, vegetables, whole grains, legumes, and nuts, you ensure an ample intake of fiber, supporting regular bowel movements, preventing constipation, and reducing the risk of digestive disorders.

2. Rich in Phytonutrients: Plant-based foods are packed with a wide array of phytonutrients, including antioxidants, polyphenols, and flavonoids. These compounds have powerful anti-inflammatory properties and help protect your gut lining from damage caused by oxidative stress. By reducing inflammation in the gut, plant-based nutrition supports a healthy gut environment, minimizing the risk of chronic diseases and promoting optimal digestion.

3. Gut Microbiota Balance: A plant-based diet can positively influence the composition and diversity of your gut microbiota. Plant foods contain prebiotics, which are indigestible fibers that serve as food for the beneficial bacteria in your gut. By nourishing these bacteria, you promote their growth and activity, creating a thriving community that supports optimal gut health. A diverse gut microbiota is associated with improved digestion, enhanced immune function, and reduced inflammation.

4. Reduced Intake of Inflammatory Foods: Animal-based products, such as red meat and processed meats, have been linked to increased inflammation in the body. By adopting a plant-based diet, you naturally reduce your intake of these inflammatory foods. Instead, you focus on consuming whole, plant-based foods that are anti-inflammatory in nature. This shift can help alleviate gut inflammation, reduce the risk of gastrointestinal disorders, and support a healthy gut environment.

5. Enhanced Nutrient Density: Plant-based foods are rich in essential nutrients, vitamins, and minerals that are vital for optimal gut health. By consuming a variety of plant foods, you ensure a diverse nutrient intake that supports the overall function of your digestive system. Nutrients like vitamin C, vitamin E, zinc, and magnesium found in plant foods play important roles in maintaining gut integrity, supporting the immune system, and promoting healthy digestion.

6. Improved Digestive Enzymes: Plant-based foods are often easier to digest compared to animal-based foods. They contain natural digestive enzymes that help break down complex carbohydrates, proteins, and fats, facilitating the digestive

process. This can alleviate the burden on your digestive system, allowing it to function more efficiently and reducing the likelihood of digestive discomfort.

<u>Debunking Common Misconceptions About Plant-Based Diets</u>

Plant-based diets have gained significant popularity in recent years, but along with that popularity comes a fair share of misconceptions. Let's debunk some of the most common misconceptions surrounding plant-based diets and shed light on the truth:

1. Lack of Protein: One of the most prevalent misconceptions is that plant-based diets lack sufficient protein. However, this couldn't be further from the truth. Plant-based sources of protein, such as legumes, tofu, tempeh, seitan, quinoa, and hemp seeds, are abundant and can provide all the essential amino acids your body needs. By incorporating a variety of plant-based protein sources into your diet, you can easily meet your protein requirements.

2. Inadequate Nutrient Intake: Another misconception is that plant-based diets are nutritionally deficient. However, with proper planning and a diverse selection of plant foods, a well-balanced plant-based diet can provide all the necessary nutrients your body needs. Plant-based foods are rich in vitamins, minerals, antioxidants, and fiber, which are essential for optimal health. It's important to pay attention to key nutrients like vitamin B12, iron, calcium, and omega-3 fatty acids, and ensure you're getting them through fortified foods or supplements if necessary.

3. Bland and Boring Food: Many people believe that plant-based diets consist of bland and tasteless food. However, plant-based cuisine is incredibly diverse and flavorful. With a wide range of herbs, spices, fruits, vegetables, whole grains, legumes, and plant-based alternatives, you can create delicious and satisfying meals. The key is to experiment with different flavors, cooking techniques, and recipes to discover the endless possibilities of plant-based cooking.

4. Difficulty Meeting Caloric Needs: Some individuals worry that it's challenging to meet their caloric needs on a plant-based diet. However, plant-based diets can be tailored to meet various caloric requirements, whether you're looking to lose weight, maintain weight, or gain muscle. Caloric needs can be met through whole plant foods like grains, legumes, nuts, seeds, and healthy fats. It's important to listen to your body's hunger and fullness cues and adjust portion sizes accordingly.

5. Limited Food Choices: A common misconception is that a plant-based diet restricts food choices. However, the reality is quite the opposite. Plant-based diets open up a world of possibilities by encouraging the consumption of a wide variety of fruits, vegetables, whole grains, legumes, nuts, seeds, herbs, and spices. This abundance of plant-based options allows for creativity in the kitchen and the opportunity to explore new flavors and textures.

6. Expensive and Inconvenient: Many people believe that following a plant-based diet is expensive and inconvenient. While it's true that some plant-based alternatives can be more expensive, a plant-based diet can also be cost-effective. Focus-

ing on whole plant foods, such as grains, legumes, and seasonal produce, can be budget-friendly. Additionally, with proper meal planning and preparation, a plant-based diet can be just as convenient as any other dietary approach.

The Basics of Gut Health

The digestive system is a marvel of intricate structures and processes that work together to break down food, absorb nutrients, and eliminate waste. Let's embark on a journey through the anatomy of the digestive system to gain a deeper understanding of its remarkable workings:

1. Mouth and Salivary Glands: The journey begins in the mouth, where digestion begins. The mouth contains teeth, which aid in mechanical digestion by breaking down food into smaller pieces. The salivary glands secrete saliva, which contains enzymes like amylase that initiate the chemical breakdown of carbohydrates. The tongue helps in swallowing and taste perception.

2. Esophagus: Once food is chewed and mixed with saliva, it travels down the esophagus, a muscular tube that connects the mouth to the stomach. The esophagus uses rhythmic contractions called peristalsis to propel the food towards the stomach.

3. Stomach: The stomach is a muscular organ that further

breaks down food through mechanical churning and chemical digestion. It secretes gastric juices, including hydrochloric acid and enzymes like pepsin, to break down proteins. The stomach also plays a role in sterilizing food by killing bacteria with its acidic environment.

4. Small Intestine: The small intestine is where most of the digestion and absorption of nutrients occur. It consists of three parts: the duodenum, jejunum, and ileum. The inner lining of the small intestine is covered in tiny finger-like projections called villi, which increase the surface area for nutrient absorption. Enzymes from the pancreas and bile from the liver aid in the breakdown of carbohydrates, proteins, and fats. Nutrients are absorbed into the bloodstream and transported to various parts of the body.

5. Liver and Gallbladder: The liver, located in the upper right portion of the abdomen, plays a crucial role in digestion. It produces bile, which is stored in the gallbladder. Bile helps in the digestion and absorption of fats by emulsifying them into smaller droplets, increasing their surface area for enzymatic action.

6. Pancreas: The pancreas, situated behind the stomach, is both an endocrine and exocrine gland. It produces digestive enzymes, such as amylase, lipase, and proteases, which are released into the small intestine to break down carbohydrates, fats, and proteins. The pancreas also produces insulin and glucagon, hormones involved in regulating blood sugar levels.

7. Large Intestine (Colon): The large intestine is responsible

for absorbing water, electrolytes, and vitamins produced by gut bacteria. It consists of the cecum, colon, rectum, and anus. The colon houses a vast community of beneficial bacteria that aid in the fermentation of indigestible carbohydrates and the production of vitamins like vitamin K and certain B vitamins. The remaining waste material is formed into feces and eliminated through the rectum and anus.

8. Rectum and Anus: The rectum serves as a temporary storage site for feces until elimination. The anus is the opening through which feces are expelled from the body during a bowel movement.

The Hidden Heroes of Digestive Health

The gut microbiota, also known as the gut microbiome, refers to the trillions of microorganisms that reside in our gastrointestinal tract. These microorganisms, including bacteria, viruses, fungi, and other microbes, play a crucial role in maintaining our overall health and well-being. Let's delve into the fascinating world of gut microbiota and uncover their essential functions:

1. Digestion and Nutrient Absorption: The gut microbiota aids in the digestion and absorption of certain nutrients that our body cannot break down on its own. They produce enzymes that help break down complex carbohydrates, such as fiber, into simpler molecules that can be absorbed by the body. Additionally, they assist in the breakdown of bile acids, which are necessary for the absorption of fats and fat-soluble vitamins.

2. Immune System Regulation: The gut microbiota plays a pivotal role in regulating our immune system. They help train and educate our immune cells, ensuring they respond appropriately to harmful pathogens while maintaining tolerance to harmless substances. A well-balanced gut microbiota promotes a healthy immune response and helps protect against autoimmune diseases, allergies, and infections.

3. Production of Vitamins and Short-Chain Fatty Acids: Certain strains of gut bacteria have the ability to produce vitamins, such as vitamin K, biotin, and folate, which are essential for various bodily functions. Additionally, the gut microbiota ferments dietary fiber and produces short-chain fatty acids (SCFAs), such as butyrate, propionate, and acetate. SCFAs provide energy to the cells lining the colon, promote a healthy gut environment, and have anti-inflammatory properties.

4. Metabolism and Weight Regulation: Emerging research suggests that the composition of the gut microbiota may influence our metabolism and weight regulation. Certain bacteria in the gut are associated with a higher efficiency in extracting energy from food, potentially leading to weight gain. Conversely, a diverse and balanced gut microbiota, achieved through a healthy diet rich in fiber and fermented foods, may support a healthy weight and metabolism.

5. Mental Health and Brain Function: The gut microbiota has a bidirectional communication pathway with the brain, known as the gut-brain axis. This communication is facilitated through various mechanisms, including the production of neurotransmitters and the influence on the immune system.

The gut microbiota has been implicated in mental health conditions such as anxiety, depression, and even neurodegenerative disorders. Maintaining a healthy gut microbiota through a balanced diet and lifestyle may positively impact mental well-being.

6. Protection Against Pathogens: A diverse and balanced gut microbiota acts as a protective barrier against harmful pathogens. The presence of beneficial bacteria prevents the colonization of pathogenic microorganisms by competing for resources and producing antimicrobial substances. This defense mechanism helps maintain a healthy gut environment and reduces the risk of infections.

7. Regulation of Intestinal Permeability: The gut microbiota plays a role in maintaining the integrity of the intestinal barrier. They help regulate the tight junctions between intestinal cells, preventing the leakage of harmful substances into the bloodstream. Disruption of the gut microbiota balance can lead to increased intestinal permeability, also known as "leaky gut," which is associated with various health conditions and chronic inflammation.

Factors Affecting Gut Health

When it comes to maintaining optimal gut health, it is essential to understand the various factors that can influence the delicate balance of our digestive system. Our gut is a complex ecosystem, and several internal and external elements can impact its functionality. In this section, we will explore some of the key factors that can affect gut health.

1. Diet:

One of the most significant factors influencing gut health is our diet. The foods we consume play a crucial role in shaping the composition and diversity of our gut microbiota. A diet high in processed foods, refined sugars, and unhealthy fats can disrupt the balance of beneficial bacteria in our gut, leading to inflammation, digestive issues, and a weakened immune system. On the other hand, a plant-based diet rich in fiber, antioxidants, and phytonutrients can promote a healthy gut environment and support the growth of beneficial bacteria.

2. Stress:

Stress, both acute and chronic, can have a profound impact on our gut health. When we experience stress, our body releases stress hormones like cortisol, which can disrupt the balance of gut bacteria and compromise the integrity of the gut lining. This can lead to increased permeability, commonly known as "leaky gut," allowing toxins and undigested food particles to enter the bloodstream and trigger inflammation. Managing stress through practices like meditation, deep breathing exercises, and engaging in activities we enjoy can help support a healthy gut.

3. Medications:

Certain medications, such as antibiotics, can have a significant impact on gut health. While antibiotics are crucial for treating bacterial infections, they can also disrupt the balance of gut bacteria by killing off both harmful and beneficial microbes. This disruption can lead to digestive issues, such as diarrhea and an overgrowth of harmful bacteria like Clostridium difficile. If you need to take antibiotics, it is essential to work with your healthcare provider to minimize their impact on gut health by considering probiotic supplementation or incorporating gut-healing foods into your diet.

4. Sleep:
Quality sleep is vital for overall health, including gut health. Poor sleep patterns or chronic sleep deprivation can disrupt the balance of gut bacteria and impair gut function. Studies have shown that sleep disturbances can lead to an increase in harmful gut bacteria and a decrease in beneficial bacteria. Aim for a consistent sleep schedule, create a relaxing bedtime routine, and prioritize getting enough restful sleep to support a healthy gut.

5. Physical Activity:
Regular physical activity not only benefits our cardiovascular health and weight management but also plays a role in maintaining a healthy gut. Exercise has been shown to increase the diversity of gut bacteria and promote the production of short-chain fatty acids, which are beneficial for gut health. Engaging in moderate-intensity activities like walking, jogging, or yoga can help support a healthy gut and overall well-being.

6. Environmental Factors:
Environmental factors, such as pollution, toxins, and exposure to certain chemicals, can also impact gut health. Prolonged exposure to environmental pollutants can disrupt the delicate balance of gut bacteria and contribute to gut inflammation. Whenever possible, try to minimize exposure to harmful environmental factors by choosing organic produce, using natural cleaning products, and reducing exposure to air pollutants.

It is important to note that while these factors can influence gut health, each person's gut microbiota is unique, and individual responses may vary. Understanding these factors and making conscious choices to support a healthy gut can go a long way in improving digestion, reducing bloating, and enhancing overall well-being.

The Fundamentals of a Plant-Based Diet

A plant-based diet is more than just a passing trend; it is a lifestyle choice rooted in the belief that the majority of our food should come from plant sources. While there are various interpretations of what a plant-based diet entails, the overarching principle remains the same: prioritizing whole, minimally processed plant foods while minimizing or eliminating the consumption of animal products.

1. Emphasis on Plants:

At the core of a plant-based diet is a strong emphasis on consuming a wide variety of plant foods. This includes fruits, vegetables, whole grains, legumes, nuts, and seeds. These plant-based foods are rich in essential nutrients, fiber, antioxidants, and phytonutrients that support overall health and well-being.

2. Minimization of Animal Products:

While a plant-based diet does not necessarily eliminate all animal products, it does prioritize minimizing their consumption. Some individuals choose to eliminate all animal products and follow a vegan diet, while others may include small amounts of animal products on occasion. The key is to shift the focus towards plant foods as the foundation of the diet.

3. Whole Foods Approach:

A plant-based diet encourages the consumption of whole, unprocessed or minimally processed foods. This means opting for whole grains instead of refined grains, choosing fresh fruits and vegetables over canned or processed ones, and preparing meals from scratch using whole ingredients whenever possible. By prioritizing whole foods, you can maximize the nutritional value of your meals and minimize the intake of additives, preservatives, and unhealthy fats.

4. Diversity and Balance:

Variety is essential in a plant-based diet to ensure you receive a wide range of nutrients. Aim to incorporate a rainbow of fruits and vegetables, different types of whole grains, a variety of legumes, and a mix of nuts and seeds into your meals. This diversity not only provides a broad spectrum of nutrients but also keeps your meals interesting and enjoyable.

5. Mindful Eating:

A plant-based diet encourages mindful eating practices, which involve being present and aware of your food choices, eating slowly, and paying attention to hunger and fullness cues. By cultivating a mindful eating approach, you can develop a healthier relationship with food, savor the flavors and textures of your meals, and make conscious choices that support your overall well-being.

6. Environmental Considerations:

Many individuals choose a plant-based diet not only for personal health reasons but also for environmental sustainability. Plant-based diets have a lower carbon footprint and require fewer natural resources compared to diets rich in animal products. By adopting a plant-based lifestyle, you can contribute to reducing greenhouse gas emissions, conserving water, and preserving biodiversity.

Understanding the Spectrum of Plant-Based Diets

While the core principle of a plant-based diet remains the same - prioritizing plant foods - there are different variations and approaches within the plant-based spectrum. These variations allow individuals to tailor their dietary choices based on personal preferences, health goals, and ethical considerations. Let's explore some of the different types of plant-based diets:

1. Vegan Diet:

A vegan diet is the most strict form of plant-based eating. It excludes all animal products, including meat, poultry, fish, dairy, eggs, and honey. Vegans rely solely on plant-based foods for their nutritional needs. This diet is often chosen for ethical reasons, as it avoids the exploitation and harm of animals.

2. Vegetarian Diet:

A vegetarian diet eliminates meat, poultry, and fish but may include other animal-derived products such as dairy, eggs, and honey. There are different types of vegetarian diets, including lacto-vegetarian (includes dairy but excludes eggs), ovo-vegetarian (includes eggs but excludes dairy), and lacto-ovo vegetarian (includes both dairy and eggs).

3. Flexitarian Diet:

The flexitarian diet, also known as semi-vegetarianism, is a flexible approach that primarily focuses on plant-based foods but allows for occasional consumption of small amounts of meat, poultry, or fish. Flexitarians typically prioritize plant foods in their meals but may choose to include animal products on special occasions or when dining out.

4. Pescatarian Diet:

A pescatarian diet is primarily plant-based but includes fish and seafood. Pescatarians exclude meat and poultry but may consume dairy, eggs, and fish for their sources of protein and essential nutrients. This diet is often chosen for its perceived health benefits and the inclusion of omega-3 fatty acids found in fish.

5. Raw Vegan Diet:

The raw vegan diet takes plant-based eating to the next level by emphasizing the consumption of raw, uncooked, and unprocessed plant foods. This diet includes fruits, vegetables, nuts, seeds, and sprouted grains. Raw food enthusiasts believe that cooking destroys enzymes and reduces the nutritional value of foods.

6. Whole Food Plant-Based Diet:

The whole food plant-based (WFPB) diet focuses on consuming whole, minimally processed plant foods while avoiding or minimizing the intake of refined grains, added sugars, and oils. This diet emphasizes whole grains, legumes, fruits, vegetables, nuts, and seeds. It promotes the consumption of nutrient-dense foods in their most natural form.

Transitioning to a Plant-Based Diet

Transitioning to a plant-based diet can be an exciting and transformative journey for your health and well-being. While it may seem daunting at first, with the right approach and mindset, you can make a successful transition. Here are some tips to help you navigate the process:

1. Educate Yourself:

Start by educating yourself about the benefits and principles of a plant-based diet. Understand the nutrients you need to focus on, the potential challenges you may face, and the variety of plant-based foods available to you. This knowledge will empower you to make informed choices and ensure you meet your nutritional needs.

2. Take it Slow:

Transitioning to a plant-based diet doesn't have to happen overnight. Consider taking a gradual approach by gradually reducing your consumption of animal products and increasing your intake of plant-based foods. This gradual transition allows your taste buds and digestive system to adapt to the changes more easily.

3. Plan Your Meals:

Meal planning is key to a successful transition. Take some time each week to plan your meals and make a grocery list. Include a variety of plant-based foods, such as fruits, vegetables, whole grains, legumes, nuts, and seeds. Experiment with new recipes and flavors to keep your meals exciting and enjoyable.

4. Focus on Whole Foods:

As you transition, prioritize whole, unprocessed or minimally processed plant foods. These foods are rich in nutrients and provide the foundation for a healthy plant-based diet. Incorporate a variety of colorful fruits and vegetables, whole grains like quinoa and brown rice, legumes like lentils and chickpeas, and healthy fats from nuts and seeds.

5. Explore Plant-Based Alternatives:

There are now numerous plant-based alternatives available for meat, dairy, and other animal products. Experiment with plant-based proteins like tofu, tempeh, seitan, and legumes. Try dairy alternatives like almond milk, coconut milk, or oat milk. These alternatives can help ease the transition and provide familiar flavors and textures.

6. Find Support:

Seek support from like-minded individuals who are also transitioning to a plant-based diet or already following one. Join online communities, attend local meetups, or find a plant-based buddy to share tips, recipes, and experiences. Having a support system can provide motivation, accountability, and a sense of belonging.

7. Listen to Your Body:

Pay attention to how your body responds to the changes. Everyone's digestive system is unique, and you may need to make adjustments along the way. If you experience any discomfort or deficiencies, consult with a healthcare professional or registered dietitian who specializes in plant-based nutrition to ensure you are meeting your nutrient needs.

8. Be Mindful of Nutrients:

While a well-planned plant-based diet can provide all the necessary nutrients, it's important to be mindful of certain nutrients that may require extra attention, such as vitamin B12, omega-3 fatty acids, iron, calcium, and vitamin D. Consider incorporating fortified foods or supplements if needed, and consult with a healthcare professional for personalized guidance.

Remember, transitioning to a plant-based diet is a personal journey, and it's important to be patient and kind to yourself throughout the process. Celebrate your progress and focus on the positive changes you are making for your health, the environment, and animal welfare.

Nutrients for Gut Health

Maintaining a healthy gut is essential for overall well-being and optimal digestion. A plant-based diet can provide a wide range of nutrients that support a thriving digestive system. Let's explore some key nutrients and their roles in gut health:

1. Fiber:

Fiber is a crucial nutrient for gut health. It adds bulk to the stool, promotes regular bowel movements, and supports the growth of beneficial gut bacteria. Plant-based foods such as fruits, vegetables, whole grains, legumes, nuts, and seeds are excellent sources of dietary fiber. Aim for a variety of fiber-rich foods to ensure you're getting both soluble and insoluble fiber.

2. Probiotics:

Probiotics are beneficial bacteria that promote a healthy balance of gut flora. They help break down food, enhance nutrient absorption, and support immune function. While probiotics are commonly associated with fermented dairy products, there are plenty of plant-based sources as well. Look for plant-based yogurts, kefir, sauerkraut, kimchi, tempeh, and miso to incorporate probiotics into your diet.

3. Prebiotics:

Prebiotics are non-digestible fibers that serve as food for probiotics, helping them thrive in the gut. They promote the growth of beneficial bacteria and contribute to a healthy gut environment. Plant-based sources of prebiotics include onions, garlic, leeks, asparagus, bananas, oats, flaxseeds, and chicory root.

4. Omega-3 Fatty Acids:

Omega-3 fatty acids have anti-inflammatory properties and play a role in maintaining a healthy gut lining. They can help reduce inflammation in the digestive tract and support overall gut health. Plant-based sources of omega-3 fatty acids include flaxseeds, chia seeds, hemp seeds, walnuts, and algae-based supplements.

5. Antioxidants:

Antioxidants help protect the cells in the gut from oxidative stress and inflammation. They can help reduce the risk of digestive disorders and support a healthy gut lining. Plant-based foods, particularly brightly colored fruits and vegetables, are rich in antioxidants. Include a variety of berries, leafy greens, bell peppers, and citrus fruits in your diet.

6. Vitamins and Minerals:

A well-rounded plant-based diet can provide all the essential vitamins and minerals necessary for gut health. Some key nutrients to pay attention to include vitamin B12, iron, calcium, zinc, magnesium, and vitamin D. While these nutrients can be obtained from plant-based sources, it's important to ensure adequate intake through fortified foods or supplements if needed.

7. Hydration:
Staying hydrated is crucial for maintaining a healthy digestive system. Water helps soften the stool, prevent constipation, and support the overall functioning of the digestive tract. Aim to drink an adequate amount of water throughout the day and include hydrating foods like fruits and vegetables in your meals.

Plant-Based Sources of Essential Nutrients
A well-planned plant-based diet can provide all the essential nutrients your body needs for optimal health. Let's explore some plant-based sources of key nutrients:

1. Protein:
Contrary to popular belief, plant-based diets can easily meet protein needs. Incorporate a variety of plant-based protein sources such as legumes (beans, lentils, chickpeas), tofu, tempeh, seitan, edamame, quinoa, hemp seeds, chia seeds, and spirulina. These foods provide all the essential amino acids necessary for a complete protein profile.

2. Calcium:
Calcium is vital for strong bones and teeth. Plant-based sources of calcium include leafy greens (kale, collard greens, spinach), broccoli, tofu (made with calcium sulfate), fortified plant-based milk (almond, soy, oat, rice), sesame seeds, tahini, and almonds. Aim to include these foods in your daily meals to meet your calcium needs.

3. Iron:

Iron is essential for oxygen transport and energy production. Plant-based sources of iron include legumes, lentils, tofu, tempeh, quinoa, fortified cereals, dark leafy greens (spinach, kale), dried fruits (apricots, raisins), pumpkin seeds, and blackstrap molasses. Enhance iron absorption by consuming vitamin C-rich foods like citrus fruits, bell peppers, and strawberries alongside iron-rich foods.

4. Omega-3 Fatty Acids:
Omega-3 fatty acids are important for heart health and brain function. Plant-based sources of omega-3s include flaxseeds, chia seeds, hemp seeds, walnuts, algae-based supplements, and seaweed. Consider incorporating these foods into your diet to ensure an adequate intake of omega-3 fatty acids.

5. Vitamin B12:
Vitamin B12 is crucial for nerve function and red blood cell production. As a plant-based eater, it's important to supplement with vitamin B12 or consume fortified foods like plant-based milk, breakfast cereals, nutritional yeast, and meat substitutes. Check labels to ensure adequate vitamin B12 intake.

6. Vitamin D:
Vitamin D is essential for bone health and immune function. While sunlight is the best source of vitamin D, plant-based sources include fortified plant-based milk, fortified orange juice, mushrooms exposed to sunlight, and supplements. Consider getting your vitamin D levels checked and consult with a healthcare professional for personalized guidance.

7. Zinc:

Zinc is important for immune function and cell growth. Plant-based sources of zinc include legumes, tofu, tempeh, seeds (pumpkin, sesame, hemp), nuts (cashews, almonds, peanuts), whole grains (quinoa, brown rice), and fortified breakfast cereals. Including a variety of these foods in your diet can help meet your zinc needs.

The Triad of Gut Health

When it comes to maintaining a healthy gut, three key players take center stage: fiber, prebiotics, and probiotics. Let's delve into the importance of each and how they work together to support your digestive system.

1. Fiber: The Gut's Best Friend

Fiber is a type of carbohydrate that cannot be digested by the human body. While it may not provide us with direct nutrients, its impact on gut health is immense. There are two types of fiber: soluble and insoluble.

Soluble fiber dissolves in water and forms a gel-like substance in the digestive tract. It helps regulate blood sugar levels, lowers cholesterol, and promotes a feeling of fullness. Good sources of soluble fiber include oats, barley, legumes, apples, citrus fruits, and flaxseeds.

Insoluble fiber, on the other hand, adds bulk to the stool and promotes regular bowel movements. It helps prevent constipation and maintains a healthy digestive system. Whole grains, vegetables, nuts, and seeds are excellent sources of insoluble fiber.

By including a variety of fiber-rich foods in your diet, you provide nourishment to the trillions of beneficial bacteria residing in your gut. These bacteria ferment the fiber, producing short-chain fatty acids (SCFAs) that provide energy for the cells lining the colon. SCFAs also have anti-inflammatory properties and support a healthy gut environment.

2. Prebiotics: Feeding the Good Bacteria

Prebiotics are non-digestible fibers that serve as food for probiotics, the beneficial bacteria in your gut. They act as a fertilizer, promoting the growth and activity of these friendly microbes. By consuming prebiotics, you create an environment in your gut that is favorable for the growth of beneficial bacteria.

Some common sources of prebiotics include onions, garlic, leeks, asparagus, bananas, oats, flaxseeds, and chicory root. Including these foods in your diet can help nourish and support the growth of probiotics, leading to a healthier gut microbiome.

3. Probiotics: The Gut's Guardians

Probiotics are live microorganisms that confer health benefits when consumed in adequate amounts. These beneficial bacteria help maintain a balanced gut microbiome, support digestion, enhance nutrient absorption, and strengthen the immune system.

While probiotics are often associated with fermented dairy products like yogurt and kefir, there are plenty of plant-based sources as well. Look for plant-based yogurts made from coconut, almond, or soy milk. Fermented foods like sauerkraut, kimchi, tempeh, and miso also contain probiotics.

Incorporating probiotic-rich foods into your diet can help replenish and diversify the beneficial bacteria in your gut. However, it's important to note that not all probiotic strains are the same, and their effectiveness may vary. Consult with a healthcare professional or registered dietitian to determine the most suitable probiotic options for your specific needs.

The synergy between fiber, prebiotics, and probiotics is crucial for maintaining a healthy gut. Fiber provides the nourishment for beneficial bacteria, prebiotics act as their food source, and probiotics help maintain a balanced gut microbiome. By incorporating a variety of fiber-rich foods, prebiotic sources, and probiotic-rich foods into your diet, you can nurture your gut and support optimal digestive health.

Healing Foods for Gut Health

A healthy gut is the foundation of overall well-being. To support your gut health, incorporating specific plant-based foods into your diet can make a significant difference. These foods are rich in fiber, prebiotics, and other beneficial compounds that nourish your gut microbiome. Let's explore some of these gut-friendly plant-based foods:

1. Fermented Foods:
Fermented foods are a fantastic addition to any gut-healthy diet. They are rich in probiotics, which help maintain a balanced gut microbiome. Some plant-based fermented foods include:

- Sauerkraut: Made from fermented cabbage, sauerkraut is packed with beneficial bacteria and enzymes that support digestion.
- Kimchi: A traditional Korean dish made from fermented vegetables, kimchi is known for its probiotic content and spicy flavor.
- Tempeh: A fermented soy product, tempeh is a great source of plant-based protein and probiotics. It has a nutty flavor and

a firm texture, making it versatile in various dishes.

2. Whole Grains:

Whole grains are excellent sources of fiber, which promotes healthy digestion and feeds beneficial gut bacteria. Incorporate the following whole grains into your diet:

- Oats: Rich in soluble fiber, oats help regulate bowel movements and support a healthy gut environment.
- Brown Rice: A fiber-rich alternative to white rice, brown rice provides nourishment to the gut microbiome.
- Quinoa: This ancient grain is not only a complete protein but also a good source of fiber, supporting gut health.

3. Legumes:

Legumes, such as beans, lentils, and chickpeas, are nutritional powerhouses that offer a host of benefits for gut health. They are high in both fiber and prebiotics, making them ideal for promoting a healthy gut microbiome. Some legumes to include in your diet are:

- Black Beans: These beans are rich in fiber and antioxidants, supporting gut health and overall well-being.
- Lentils: Packed with fiber and protein, lentils are a versatile legume that can be added to soups, salads, and stews.
- Chickpeas: Known for their role in hummus, chickpeas are a great source of fiber and prebiotics, nourishing your gut microbiome.

4. Leafy Greens:

Leafy greens are not only nutrient-dense but also beneficial for gut health. They contain fiber, antioxidants, and other compounds that support a healthy digestive system. Some gut-friendly leafy greens include:

- Spinach: Rich in fiber and antioxidants, spinach helps promote regular bowel movements and supports gut health.
  - Kale: Packed with vitamins, minerals, and fiber, kale is a nutritional powerhouse that nourishes your gut microbiome.
  - Swiss Chard: This leafy green is high in fiber and contains a variety of antioxidants that support gut health.

5. Berries:

Berries are not only delicious but also offer numerous health benefits, including promoting gut health. They are packed with fiber, antioxidants, and other compounds that support a healthy gut microbiome. Some gut-friendly berries include:

- Blueberries: Known for their high antioxidant content, blueberries also provide fiber to support a healthy gut.
  - Raspberries: These berries are rich in fiber and polyphenols, which have been linked to improved gut health.
  - Strawberries: Packed with vitamins, minerals, and fiber, strawberries are a tasty addition to a gut-healthy diet.

Unleashing the Magic of Fermentation

Fermentation is an ancient preservation technique that has been used for centuries to transform food and beverages. Beyond preservation, fermentation offers a myriad of benefits for our health, particularly when it comes to our gut. In this chapter, we will explore the fascinating world of fermented foods and uncover the numerous advantages they provide.

1. Enhanced Digestion and Nutrient Absorption

One of the primary benefits of fermented foods is their ability to enhance digestion and improve nutrient absorption. During the fermentation process, beneficial bacteria, yeasts, or fungi convert carbohydrates into organic acids and gases. These organic acids, such as lactic acid, help break down food, making it easier for our bodies to digest.

Additionally, fermentation increases the bioavailability of nutrients in the food. For example, fermented dairy products like yogurt and kefir contain enzymes that break down lactose, making them more tolerable for individuals with lactose intolerance. Fermented foods also increase the levels of certain vitamins, such as B vitamins and vitamin K2, which are produced by the beneficial bacteria during fermentation.

2. Gut Health and Microbiome Balance

Fermented foods are rich in probiotics, which are beneficial bacteria that support a healthy gut microbiome. These probiotics help restore and maintain a balanced microbial community in our digestive system. A diverse and thriving gut microbiome is essential for optimal digestion, nutrient absorption, immune function, and overall well-being.

Consuming fermented foods regularly can help populate the gut with beneficial bacteria, improving the diversity and abundance of microbial species. This, in turn, supports a healthy gut environment and reduces the risk of digestive issues such as bloating, gas, and constipation.

3. Immune System Support

The gut plays a crucial role in our immune system, and fermented foods can help strengthen our body's defense mechanisms. Approximately 70% of our immune cells reside in the gut, and a healthy gut microbiome is essential for proper immune function.

The probiotics found in fermented foods stimulate the production of immune-boosting compounds and help regulate the immune response. They also compete with harmful bacteria for resources and space in the gut, preventing the overgrowth of pathogens.

4. Improved Mental Health

Emerging research suggests a strong connection between the gut and the brain, known as the gut-brain axis. The gut microbiome produces neurotransmitters and communicates with the brain through various pathways, influencing our mood, emotions, and mental health.

Consuming fermented foods may have a positive impact on mental well-being. Probiotics in fermented foods can modulate neurotransmitter production, reduce inflammation, and improve the gut-brain communication. This may help alleviate symptoms of anxiety, depression, and stress.

5. Enhanced Nutritional Value

Fermentation not only enhances digestion and nutrient absorption but also increases the nutritional value of certain foods. For example, fermented vegetables like sauerkraut and kimchi have higher levels of vitamins, minerals, and antioxidants compared to their raw counterparts. Fermentation breaks down complex compounds, making them more bioavailable and easier for our bodies to utilize.

Incorporating Fermented Foods into Your Diet

To reap the benefits of fermented foods, consider adding the following options to your diet:

- Yogurt: Choose plain, unsweetened yogurt with live and active cultures. Avoid varieties with added sugars or artificial flavors.

- Kefir: A fermented milk drink, kefir is rich in probiotics and can be enjoyed on its own or added to smoothies.

- Sauerkraut: Made from fermented cabbage, sauerkraut is a tangy and crunchy addition to sandwiches, salads, or as a side dish.

- Kimchi: A Korean staple, kimchi is a spicy fermented vegetable dish that adds a flavorful kick to stir-fries, rice bowls, and more.

- Tempeh: A fermented soy product, tempeh is a versatile meat substitute that can be grilled, stir-fried, or added to sandwiches and salads.

- Miso: A traditional Japanese seasoning made from fermented soybeans, miso adds depth of flavor to soups, marinades, and dressings.

Remember to choose high-quality, organic options whenever possible to ensure the best quality and nutritional value.

<u>Introduction to Gut-Healthy Plant-Based Eating</u>

Maintaining a gut-healthy plant-based diet doesn't have to be boring or restrictive. In fact, there are countless delicious and nourishing recipes that can support your gut health while satisfying your taste buds. Whether you're a seasoned plant-based eater or just starting to explore this lifestyle, these 20 recipes and meal ideas will help you create a diverse and gut-friendly menu.

1. Breakfast Options:

Gut-Healing Smoothie Bowl

Prep Time: 10 minutes
   Serving: 1

Ingredients:
   - 1 cup spinach
   - 1/2 cup frozen berries (such as blueberries, raspberries, or strawberries)
   - 1/2 cup almond milk (or any plant-based milk of your choice)
   - 1 tablespoon chia seeds
   - 1 scoop plant-based protein powder
   - Toppings: sliced banana, granola, coconut yogurt

Instructions:
   1. In a blender, combine the spinach, frozen berries, almond milk, chia seeds, and plant-based protein powder.
   2. Blend on high until smooth and creamy. If the mixture is too thick, you can add a little more almond milk to reach your

desired consistency.

3. Pour the smoothie into a bowl.

4. Top with sliced banana, a sprinkle of granola, and a dollop of coconut yogurt.

5. Feel free to get creative with additional toppings like nuts, seeds, or a drizzle of honey if desired.

6. Serve immediately and enjoy!

This Gut-Healing Smoothie Bowl is packed with nutrients, fiber, and gut-friendly ingredients like spinach and chia seeds. It's a delicious and nourishing way to start your day and support your digestive health.

Overnight Chia Pudding
Prep Time: 5 minutes (plus overnight chilling)
Serving: 1

Ingredients:
- 1/4 cup chia seeds
- 1 cup almond milk (or any plant-based milk of your choice)
- 1 tablespoon maple syrup (or sweetener of your choice)
- Optional toppings: fresh berries, chopped nuts, cinnamon

Instructions:
1. In a jar or bowl, combine the chia seeds, almond milk, and maple syrup.

2. Stir well to ensure the chia seeds are evenly distributed and not clumping together.

3. Cover the jar or bowl and refrigerate overnight or for at least 4-6 hours. This will allow the chia seeds to absorb the liquid and create a pudding-like consistency.

4. The next morning, give the chia pudding a good stir to break up any clumps.

5. If desired, add your favorite toppings such as fresh berries, chopped nuts, or a sprinkle of cinnamon.

6. Enjoy the chia pudding chilled and savor its creamy texture and subtle sweetness.

This Overnight Chia Pudding is not only delicious but also a great source of fiber, omega-3 fatty acids, and plant-based protein. It's a convenient make-ahead breakfast option that will keep you satisfied and energized throughout the morning.

2. Lunch Ideas:

Gut-Nourishing Salad
  Prep Time: 15 minutes
  Serving: 2

Ingredients:
  - 4 cups mixed greens (such as spinach, kale, or arugula)
  - 1 cup roasted sweet potatoes, cubed
  - 1/2 cup cooked quinoa
  - 1/2 cup chickpeas, rinsed and drained
  - 1/4 cup sliced cucumber
  - 1/4 cup sliced radishes
  - Optional toppings: sauerkraut, pickles
  - For the Lemon-Tahini Dressing:
  - 2 tablespoons tahini
  - 2 tablespoons fresh lemon juice
  - 1 tablespoon olive oil
  - 1 teaspoon maple syrup

- Salt and pepper to taste

Instructions:

1. In a large bowl, combine the mixed greens, roasted sweet potatoes, cooked quinoa, chickpeas, sliced cucumber, and sliced radishes.

2. Toss the ingredients gently to mix them together.

3. In a separate small bowl, whisk together the tahini, fresh lemon juice, olive oil, maple syrup, salt, and pepper until well combined. Adjust the seasonings to taste.

4. Drizzle the lemon-tahini dressing over the salad and toss to coat the ingredients evenly.

5. If desired, add a spoonful of sauerkraut or pickles for an extra gut-friendly boost and tangy flavor.

6. Divide the salad into two serving bowls.

7. Serve immediately and enjoy the gut-nourishing goodness!

This Gut-Nourishing Salad is packed with fiber, vitamins, and minerals from the mixed greens, sweet potatoes, quinoa, and chickpeas. The lemon-tahini dressing adds a tangy and creamy element to tie all the flavors together.

Gut-Healthy Buddha Bowl
  Prep Time: 20 minutes
  Serving: 2

Ingredients:
  - 1 cup cooked quinoa or brown rice
  - 1 cup steamed broccoli florets
  - 1 cup roasted tofu or tempeh, cubed
  - 1 cup colorful vegetables (such as bell peppers, carrots, or

snap peas), sliced
  - 1 tablespoon grated ginger
  - 2 cloves garlic, minced
  - 2 tablespoons tamari sauce (or soy sauce)
  - Optional toppings: sesame seeds, sliced green onions

Instructions:
1. In a large skillet or wok, heat a tablespoon of oil over medium heat.

2. Add the grated ginger and minced garlic to the skillet and sauté for a minute until fragrant.

3. Add the colorful vegetables to the skillet and stir-fry for about 3-4 minutes until they are slightly tender but still crisp.

4. Push the vegetables to one side of the skillet and add the roasted tofu or tempeh to the other side. Cook for another 2-3 minutes to warm it up.

5. Drizzle the tamari sauce over the vegetables and tofu/tempeh. Toss everything together to coat evenly.

6. Divide the cooked quinoa or brown rice into two serving bowls.

7. Top each bowl with the stir-fried vegetables and tofu/tempeh mixture.

8. If desired, sprinkle sesame seeds and sliced green onions on top for added flavor and crunch.

9. Serve the Gut-Healthy Buddha Bowl immediately and enjoy the nourishing combination of flavors and textures.

This Gut-Healthy Buddha Bowl is a satisfying and nutrient-packed meal that combines whole grains, protein-rich tofu or tempeh, and a variety of colorful vegetables. The ginger and tamari sauce add a delicious umami flavor that ties everything together.

3. Snack Time:
   Gut-Friendly Trail Mix
   Prep Time: 5 minutes
   Serving: 4

Ingredients:
   - 1 cup raw almonds
   - 1 cup pumpkin seeds
   - 1 cup dried cranberries
   - 1/2 cup unsweetened coconut flakes
   - 1/2 cup dark chocolate chips (at least 70% cocoa)
   - 1/4 teaspoon sea salt

Instructions:
   1. In a large bowl, combine the raw almonds, pumpkin seeds, dried cranberries, unsweetened coconut flakes, dark chocolate chips, and sea salt.
   2. Toss the ingredients together until they are well mixed.
   3. Divide the trail mix into individual serving-sized portions or store in an airtight container for later use.
   4. Enjoy the Gut-Friendly Trail Mix as a convenient and nutritious snack on-the-go or as a topping for yogurt, smoothie bowls, or salads.

This Gut-Friendly Trail Mix is packed with gut-friendly ingredients like almonds, pumpkin seeds, and dried cranberries. The combination of crunchy nuts, seeds, and sweet dried fruit creates a satisfying and nutrient-dense snack that supports gut health.

Crunchy Roasted Chickpeas
   Prep Time: 5 minutes
   Cook Time: 40 minutes
   Serving: 4

Ingredients:
   - 2 cans (15 ounces each) chickpeas (garbanzo beans), drained
and rinsed
   - 2 tablespoons olive oil
   - 1 teaspoon ground cumin
   - 1 teaspoon smoked paprika
   - 1/2 teaspoon garlic powder
   - 1/2 teaspoon sea salt
   - Optional: pinch of cayenne pepper for added heat

Instructions:
   1. Preheat your oven to 400°F (200°C).
   2. Drain and rinse the chickpeas thoroughly, then pat them
dry with a clean kitchen towel or paper towels.
   3. In a bowl, combine the chickpeas, olive oil, ground cumin,
smoked paprika, garlic powder, sea salt, and cayenne pepper (if
desired). Toss well to ensure the chickpeas are evenly coated
with the spices and oil.
   4. Spread the seasoned chickpeas in a single layer on a baking
sheet lined with parchment paper.
   5. Roast the chickpeas in the preheated oven for 35-40
minutes, or until they become golden brown and crispy. Shake
the baking sheet or stir the chickpeas halfway through the
cooking time to ensure even browning.
   6. Once roasted, remove the chickpeas from the oven and let
them cool completely before serving.

7. Enjoy the Crunchy Roasted Chickpeas as a healthy and flavorful snack on their own or as a crunchy topping for salads, soups, or Buddha bowls.

These Crunchy Roasted Chickpeas are a delicious and nutritious alternative to traditional snacks. Packed with fiber, protein, and a variety of spices, they offer a satisfying crunch and can be customized with different seasonings to suit your taste preferences.

4. Dinner Delights:
Gut-Healing Lentil Soup

Prep Time: 10 minutes
Cook Time: 40 minutes
Serving: 6

Ingredients:
- 1 cup dried lentils, rinsed and drained
- 1 tablespoon olive oil
- 1 onion, diced
- 2 carrots, diced
- 2 celery stalks, diced
- 3 cloves garlic, minced
- 1 teaspoon ground cumin
- 1 teaspoon ground turmeric
- 1/2 teaspoon ground ginger
- 1/2 teaspoon paprika
- 6 cups vegetable broth
- 1 bay leaf

- Salt and pepper to taste
- Fresh parsley, chopped (for garnish)

Instructions:
  1. In a large pot, heat the olive oil over medium heat.
  2. Add the diced onion, carrots, and celery to the pot. Sauté for about 5 minutes until the vegetables start to soften.
  3. Add the minced garlic, ground cumin, ground turmeric, ground ginger, and paprika to the pot. Stir well to coat the vegetables in the spices and cook for an additional minute.
  4. Add the rinsed lentils, vegetable broth, and bay leaf to the pot. Stir to combine.
  5. Bring the soup to a boil, then reduce the heat to low and cover the pot. Let the soup simmer for about 30-35 minutes, or until the lentils are tender.
  6. Remove the bay leaf from the soup and season with salt and pepper to taste.
  7. Ladle the Gut-Healing Lentil Soup into bowls and garnish with fresh chopped parsley.
  8. Serve the soup hot and enjoy its nourishing and comforting qualities.

This Gut-Healing Lentil Soup is not only delicious but also packed with fiber, plant-based protein, and gut-friendly ingredients. The combination of lentils, vegetables, and spices creates a flavorful and nutritious soup that supports gut health and overall well-being.

Gut-Nourishing Stir-Fry
  Prep Time: 15 minutes
  Cook Time: 10 minutes

Serving: 4

Ingredients:
- 2 tablespoons olive oil
- 1 onion, thinly sliced
- 2 cloves garlic, minced
- 1 red bell pepper, thinly sliced
- 1 yellow bell pepper, thinly sliced
- 2 cups broccoli florets
- 1 cup snap peas, trimmed
- 1 cup sliced mushrooms
- 1 cup firm tofu, cubed
- 2 tablespoons tamari sauce (or soy sauce)
- 1 tablespoon rice vinegar
- 1 teaspoon grated ginger
- 1 teaspoon sesame oil
- Optional toppings: sesame seeds, sliced green onions

Instructions:
1. In a large skillet or wok, heat the olive oil over medium heat.

2. Add the sliced onion and minced garlic to the skillet. Sauté for 2-3 minutes until the onion becomes translucent and fragrant.

3. Add the sliced bell peppers, broccoli florets, snap peas, and mushrooms to the skillet. Stir-fry for about 5 minutes until the vegetables are tender-crisp.

4. Push the vegetables to one side of the skillet and add the cubed tofu to the other side. Cook for another 2-3 minutes to warm up the tofu.

5. In a small bowl, whisk together the tamari sauce, rice

vinegar, grated ginger, and sesame oil. Pour the sauce over the stir-fry and toss everything together to coat evenly.

6. Cook for an additional minute to allow the flavors to meld together.

7. Remove the skillet from heat and sprinkle sesame seeds and sliced green onions on top if desired.

8. Serve the Gut-Nourishing Stir-Fry hot and enjoy its vibrant colors and flavors.

This Gut-Nourishing Stir-Fry is a nutrient-packed dish that combines a variety of colorful vegetables, protein-rich tofu, and a flavorful sauce. The combination of fresh ingredients and Asian-inspired flavors makes it a delicious and gut-nourishing meal option.

5. Dessert Treats:
Gut-Friendly Berry Crumble
Prep Time: 15 minutes
Cook Time: 30 minutes
Total Time: 45 minutes
Serving: 6 servings

Ingredients:
- 4 cups mixed fresh or frozen berries (such as blueberries, raspberries, and strawberries)
- 2 tablespoons maple syrup
- 1 tablespoon lemon juice
- 1 cup rolled oats
- 1/2 cup almond flour
- 1/4 cup coconut oil, melted
- 1/4 cup chopped nuts (such as almonds or walnuts)

- 2 tablespoons coconut sugar or brown sugar
- 1 teaspoon cinnamon
- Pinch of salt

Instructions:

1. Preheat your oven to 350°F (175°C). Grease a baking dish with coconut oil or use a non-stick cooking spray.

2. In a mixing bowl, combine the mixed berries, maple syrup, and lemon juice. Toss gently to coat the berries evenly with the sweetener. Transfer the berry mixture to the greased baking dish, spreading it out evenly.

3. In a separate bowl, combine the rolled oats, almond flour, melted coconut oil, chopped nuts, coconut sugar or brown sugar, cinnamon, and a pinch of salt. Mix well until the ingredients are evenly combined and form a crumbly texture.

4. Sprinkle the oat mixture evenly over the berries in the baking dish, covering them completely.

5. Place the baking dish in the preheated oven and bake for approximately 30 minutes, or until the berry mixture is bubbling and the crumble topping turns golden brown.

6. Once baked, remove the crumble from the oven and let it cool for a few minutes before serving.

7. Serve the gut-friendly berry crumble warm as is or with a dollop of coconut yogurt or dairy-free ice cream for added

creaminess.

This gut-friendly berry crumble is a delightful and nutritious dessert option that combines the natural sweetness of mixed berries with a crunchy oat and nut topping. It's rich in fiber, antioxidants, and healthy fats, making it a perfect guilt-free treat for your gut and taste buds.

Chocolate Avocado Mousse
   Prep Time: 10 minutes
   Chill Time: 1 hour
   Total Time: 1 hour 10 minutes
   Serving: 4 servings

Ingredients:
   - 2 ripe avocados
   - 1/4 cup cocoa powder
   - 1/4 cup maple syrup or agave nectar
   - 1/4 cup almond milk or any plant-based milk
   - 1 teaspoon vanilla extract
   - Optional toppings: fresh berries, shredded coconut, chopped nuts

Instructions:

1. Cut the avocados in half, remove the pits, and scoop out the flesh into a blender or food processor.

2. Add the cocoa powder, maple syrup or agave nectar, almond milk, and vanilla extract to the blender or food processor with the avocado.

3. Blend the mixture until smooth and creamy, scraping down the sides as needed to ensure everything is well combined.

4. Once the mixture is smooth, taste and adjust the sweetness if desired by adding more maple syrup or agave nectar.

5. Transfer the chocolate avocado mousse into individual serving bowls or glasses.

6. Cover the bowls or glasses with plastic wrap and refrigerate for at least 1 hour to allow the mousse to chill and set.

7. Before serving, you can garnish the mousse with fresh berries, shredded coconut, or chopped nuts for added texture and flavor.

8. Serve the chocolate avocado mousse chilled and enjoy its rich and indulgent taste.

This chocolate avocado mousse is a decadent and creamy dessert that is not only delicious but also packed with healthy fats from the avocado. Avocados are a great source of monounsaturated fats, fiber, and various vitamins and minerals, making them a nourishing addition to your gut-healthy plant-based diet.

Feel free to customize this recipe by adding a pinch of sea salt or a dash of cinnamon for extra flavor. You can also experiment with different toppings such as sliced bananas, cacao nibs, or a drizzle of nut butter.

Incorporating these recipes and meal ideas into your gut-healthy plant-based diet will not only support your digestive health but also provide you with a wide range of nutrients, flavors, and textures. Enjoy the journey of nourishing your gut and exploring the delicious possibilities of plant-based eating.

Lifestyle Factors for Gut Health

When it comes to maintaining a healthy gut, it's not just about what you eat. Other lifestyle factors, such as stress levels, quality of sleep, and regular exercise, also play a significant role in supporting optimal gut health. In this chapter, we will explore the impact of stress, sleep, and exercise on gut health and provide insights into how you can optimize these areas to promote a thriving gut ecosystem.

Stress and Gut Health

Stress can have a profound impact on the health of your gut. When you experience stress, your body releases stress hormones like cortisol, which can disrupt the balance of bacteria in your gut and compromise its integrity. This imbalance can lead to digestive issues, inflammation, and a weakened immune system.

Sleep and Gut Health

Quality sleep is essential for overall health, including gut health. During sleep, your body undergoes important restorative processes, including the repair and regeneration of cells in your gut lining. Lack of sleep or poor sleep quality can disrupt these processes and negatively impact gut health.

Exercise and Gut Health

Regular exercise not only benefits your physical fitness but also plays a crucial role in supporting gut health. Exercise helps stimulate the muscles in your digestive tract, promoting healthy digestion and regular bowel movements. It also enhances blood flow to the gut, which can improve nutrient absorption and support a diverse and balanced gut microbiome.

Practical Tips for Managing Stress and Improving Sleep

In order to support your gut health and overall well-being, it's important to effectively manage stress levels and prioritize quality sleep. In this chapter, we will provide you with practical tips and strategies to help you manage stress and improve your sleep, ultimately promoting a healthier gut and a more balanced lifestyle.

Stress Management Tips

1. Practice Mindfulness: Engage in mindfulness techniques such as meditation, deep breathing exercises, or yoga. These practices can help calm your mind, reduce stress, and promote a sense of relaxation.

2. Prioritize Self-Care: Set aside time each day for activities that bring you joy and relaxation. This could include reading, taking a bath, listening to music, or engaging in hobbies that you enjoy. Taking care of yourself is essential for managing stress.

3. Establish Boundaries: Learn to say no when you feel

overwhelmed or stretched too thin. Setting boundaries and prioritizing your own needs will help reduce stress and create a healthier balance in your life.

4. Stay Active: Regular physical activity can help reduce stress levels. Find activities that you enjoy, such as walking, jogging, dancing, or practicing yoga. Aim for at least 30 minutes of exercise most days of the week.

5. Connect with Others: Social support is crucial for managing stress. Reach out to friends, family, or support groups to share your feelings and experiences. Connecting with others can provide a sense of belonging and help alleviate stress.

Sleep Improvement Tips

1. Establish a Bedtime Routine: Create a relaxing routine before bed to signal to your body that it's time to wind down. This could include activities such as reading a book, taking a warm bath, or practicing gentle stretching or meditation.

2. Create a Sleep-Friendly Environment: Make sure your bedroom is dark, quiet, and at a comfortable temperature. Use blackout curtains, earplugs, or a white noise machine if needed. Invest in a comfortable mattress and pillows that support good sleep posture.

3. Limit Screen Time Before Bed: Avoid electronic devices, such as smartphones, tablets, or laptops, at least an hour before bedtime. The blue light emitted by these devices can interfere with your sleep-wake cycle. Instead, engage in relaxing activities or read a book.

4. Stick to a Consistent Sleep Schedule: Try to go to bed and wake up at the same time every day, even on weekends. This helps regulate your body's internal clock and promotes better sleep quality.

5. Create a Relaxing Sleep Environment: Use calming scents, such as lavender, in your bedroom. Consider using essential oils or a diffuser to create a soothing atmosphere. Experiment with relaxation techniques, such as progressive muscle relaxation or guided imagery, to help you drift off to sleep.

The Benefits of Regular Physical Activity for Gut Health

Regular physical activity is not only essential for maintaining overall health and fitness but also plays a significant role in supporting a healthy gut. In this chapter, we will explore the numerous benefits of regular physical activity for gut health and provide insights into how exercise can contribute to a thriving gut ecosystem.

Improved Digestion and Bowel Regularity

Engaging in regular physical activity can help improve digestion and promote bowel regularity. Exercise stimulates the muscles in your digestive tract, aiding in the movement of food through your system. This can help prevent constipation and promote healthy bowel movements, reducing the risk of digestive issues such as bloating and discomfort.

Enhanced Gut Microbiome Diversity

The gut microbiome refers to the trillions of microorganisms that reside in your digestive system. A diverse and balanced gut microbiome is crucial for optimal gut health. Regular physical activity has been shown to positively influence the diversity of gut bacteria, promoting a healthier gut microbiome.

Reduced Inflammation

Chronic inflammation in the gut can contribute to various digestive disorders and compromise gut health. Regular physical activity has been found to help reduce inflammation in the body, including the gut. Exercise can lower levels of inflammatory markers and promote a more balanced immune response, supporting a healthier gut environment.

Enhanced Nutrient Absorption

Regular physical activity can improve blood flow to the gut, enhancing nutrient absorption. When blood flow increases, nutrients from the food you consume are more efficiently transported to the cells in your gut lining. This can support optimal nutrient absorption and overall gut health.

Weight Management

Maintaining a healthy weight is important for gut health. Regular physical activity can help manage weight by burning calories and promoting fat loss. Excess weight, especially around the abdomen, has been linked to an increased risk of gut-related conditions. By engaging in regular exercise, you can support a healthy weight and reduce the risk of gut-related issues.

To reap the benefits of physical activity for gut health, aim for at least 150 minutes of moderate-intensity aerobic exercise or 75 minutes of vigorous-intensity aerobic exercise per week. Additionally, incorporate strength training exercises at least two days a week to build muscle and support overall fitness.

Find activities that you enjoy, such as walking, jogging, swimming, cycling, or dancing. Make physical activity a regular part of your routine by scheduling it into your day and finding ways to stay motivated, such as exercising with a friend or joining a fitness class.

Troubleshooting Digestive Issues

Digestive problems such as bloating, gas, constipation, and indigestion can be uncomfortable and disruptive to our daily lives. In this chapter, we will address these common digestive issues and provide practical tips and strategies to help alleviate symptoms and promote a healthier digestive system.

Bloating

Bloating is a sensation of fullness and tightness in the abdomen, often accompanied by visible swelling. It can be caused by various factors, including overeating, eating too quickly, consuming gas-producing foods, or underlying digestive conditions. Here are some tips to help reduce bloating:

- Eat smaller, more frequent meals to avoid overloading your digestive system.
  - Chew your food thoroughly and eat slowly to aid digestion.
  - Avoid carbonated drinks and minimize consumption of gas-producing foods such as beans, lentils, broccoli, cabbage, and onions.
  - Stay hydrated and drink plenty of water throughout the day.
  - Consider incorporating gut-friendly foods such as ginger,

peppermint, and fennel into your diet, as they may help alleviate bloating.

Gas

Excessive gas can lead to discomfort, bloating, and embarrassment. It is often caused by swallowing air while eating or drinking, consuming gas-producing foods, or an imbalance in the gut microbiome. Here are some tips to reduce gas:

- Eat slowly and avoid talking while eating to minimize swallowing air.
- Identify and limit consumption of gas-producing foods such as beans, lentils, onions, garlic, carbonated drinks, and certain vegetables like cabbage and broccoli.
- Consider incorporating probiotic-rich foods or supplements into your diet to promote a healthy gut microbiome.
- Engage in regular physical activity to help stimulate digestion and reduce gas buildup.

Constipation

Constipation is characterized by infrequent bowel movements or difficulty passing stools. It can be caused by factors such as a lack of fiber in the diet, dehydration, sedentary lifestyle, or certain medications. Here are some tips to help relieve constipation:

- Increase your fiber intake by consuming more fruits, vegetables, whole grains, and legumes.
- Stay hydrated and drink plenty of water throughout the day.
- Engage in regular physical activity to stimulate bowel movements.

- Establish a consistent bathroom routine and take your time when using the toilet.

- Consider incorporating natural laxatives such as prunes, flaxseeds, or psyllium husk into your diet, under the guidance of a healthcare professional.

Indigestion

Indigestion, also known as dyspepsia, refers to discomfort or pain in the upper abdomen, often accompanied by symptoms such as bloating, nausea, and heartburn. It can be caused by overeating, eating too quickly, consuming fatty or spicy foods, or underlying digestive conditions. Here are some tips to help manage indigestion:

- Eat smaller, more frequent meals to avoid overloading your digestive system.

- Avoid trigger foods such as fatty or spicy foods, caffeine, and alcohol.

- Practice mindful eating by chewing your food thoroughly and eating slowly.

- Consider incorporating gut-soothing foods such as ginger, chamomile, or papaya into your diet.

- If indigestion persists or worsens, consult with a healthcare professional for further evaluation and guidance.

Natural Remedies and Strategies for Alleviating Digestive Issues

When it comes to addressing digestive issues, many people prefer natural remedies and strategies that can help alleviate symptoms without relying on medication. In this chapter, we will explore a range of natural remedies and strategies that can support a healthy digestive system and provide relief from common digestive problems.

Herbal Teas for Digestive Health

Herbal teas have long been used to soothe and support digestive health. Here are some herbal teas that can help alleviate digestive issues:

1. Peppermint Tea: Peppermint has been shown to relax the muscles of the gastrointestinal tract, reducing symptoms of bloating, gas, and indigestion.

2. Ginger Tea: Ginger has anti-inflammatory properties and can help relieve nausea, bloating, and indigestion. It also aids in digestion by increasing the production of digestive enzymes.

3. Chamomile Tea: Chamomile has calming properties that can help reduce stress and promote relaxation. It can soothe the digestive system and alleviate symptoms of indigestion and bloating.

Probiotics for Gut Health

Probiotics are beneficial bacteria that can support a healthy gut microbiome. They can be found in certain foods or taken as supplements. Here are some natural sources of probiotics:

1. Yogurt: Choose plain, unsweetened yogurt that contains live

and active cultures. These cultures can help restore the balance of bacteria in the gut.

2. Kefir: Kefir is a fermented milk drink that is rich in probiotics. It can help improve digestion and promote a healthy gut microbiome.

3. Sauerkraut: Sauerkraut is fermented cabbage that contains probiotics. It can aid in digestion and support a healthy gut.

Dietary Modifications for Digestive Health

Making certain dietary modifications can also help alleviate digestive issues. Here are some strategies to consider:

1. Increase Fiber Intake: Consuming an adequate amount of fiber can promote regular bowel movements and prevent constipation. Include fruits, vegetables, whole grains, and legumes in your diet.

2. Stay Hydrated: Drinking enough water is essential for maintaining proper digestion and preventing constipation. Aim to drink at least 8 glasses of water per day.

3. Avoid Trigger Foods: Certain foods can trigger digestive issues in some individuals. Pay attention to your body and identify any foods that worsen your symptoms. Common triggers include spicy foods, fatty foods, caffeine, and alcohol.

When to Seek Professional Help for Persistent Gut Health Problems

While many digestive issues can be managed with natural remedies and lifestyle modifications, there are times when it is necessary to seek professional help. Persistent gut health problems may indicate underlying conditions that require medical attention. In this chapter, we will discuss when it is appropriate to seek professional help for digestive issues.

Red Flags to Look Out For

Certain symptoms and situations should prompt you to seek medical advice for your gut health problems. Here are some red flags to be aware of:

1. Persistent or Worsening Symptoms: If your digestive symptoms persist or worsen despite trying natural remedies and lifestyle modifications, it is important to consult with a healthcare professional. This could indicate an underlying condition that requires further evaluation and treatment.

2. Unexplained Weight Loss: If you experience unexplained weight loss along with digestive issues, it is essential to seek medical attention. Unintentional weight loss can be a sign of a more serious underlying condition.

3. Blood in Stool: The presence of blood in your stool should never be ignored. It can indicate various gastrointestinal conditions, including ulcers, hemorrhoids, or even colorectal cancer. Seek immediate medical attention if you notice blood in your stool.

4. Severe Abdominal Pain: Intense or persistent abdominal pain

that is interfering with your daily life should not be ignored. It could be a sign of a more serious condition, such as appendicitis, gallstones, or inflammatory bowel disease.

5. Difficulty Swallowing: If you experience difficulty swallowing, it is important to seek medical evaluation. This could be a symptom of an esophageal disorder or other underlying issues.

When to Consult a Healthcare Professional

In addition to the red flags mentioned above, there are certain situations where it is advisable to consult a healthcare professional for your gut health problems. These include:

1. Chronic Digestive Issues: If you have been experiencing chronic digestive issues for an extended period, it is recommended to seek medical advice. Chronic conditions such as irritable bowel syndrome (IBS), Crohn's disease, or celiac disease may require specialized treatment and management.

2. Family History of Digestive Disorders: If you have a family history of digestive disorders, it is important to discuss your symptoms with a healthcare professional. Some gastrointestinal conditions have a genetic component, and early detection and intervention can be crucial.

3. Impact on Quality of Life: If your gut health problems are significantly impacting your quality of life, it is essential to seek professional help. Digestive issues that interfere with daily activities, work, or social interactions should not be ignored.

4. Recurring Infections: If you experience recurring gastrointestinal infections, such as bacterial or parasitic infections, it is important to consult with a healthcare professional. They can help identify the underlying cause and provide appropriate treatment.

While natural remedies and lifestyle modifications can often alleviate digestive issues, there are instances where seeking professional help is necessary. Persistent or worsening symptoms, unexplained weight loss, blood in stool, severe abdominal pain, difficulty swallowing, chronic digestive issues, family history of digestive disorders, impact on quality of life, and recurring infections are all valid reasons to consult a healthcare professional. Remember, early detection and intervention can lead to better outcomes and improved gut health.

Gut Health and Overall Well-Being

The gut is often referred to as the "second brain" due to its intricate connection with various aspects of our well-being. Emerging research suggests that the health of our gut plays a significant role in not only our digestive system but also our mental health, immune function, and overall well-being. In this chapter, we will explore the fascinating connection between gut health and other aspects of well-being.

Gut Health and Mental Health

The gut-brain axis is a bidirectional communication system between the gut and the brain. The state of our gut health can influence our mental health and vice versa. Here are a few key points to consider:

1. Gut Microbiota and Mental Health: The gut is home to trillions of bacteria, collectively known as the gut microbiota. These bacteria play a crucial role in the production of neuro-transmitters such as serotonin, which is often referred to as the "feel-good" hormone. Imbalances in the gut microbiota have been linked to mental health conditions such as anxiety,

depression, and even neurodegenerative disorders.

2. Inflammation and Mental Health: Chronic inflammation in the gut can lead to increased permeability of the intestinal lining, allowing toxins and bacteria to enter the bloodstream. This condition, known as leaky gut syndrome, has been associated with increased inflammation throughout the body, including the brain. Inflammation in the brain has been linked to various mental health disorders.

3. The Role of Serotonin: As mentioned earlier, serotonin is a neurotransmitter that plays a crucial role in regulating mood. Interestingly, around 90% of serotonin is produced in the gut. A healthy gut microbiota is essential for optimal serotonin production, which can positively impact mental well-being.

Gut Health and Immune Function

The gut also plays a vital role in supporting a healthy immune system. Here's how gut health and immune function are interconnected:

1. Gut Microbiota and Immunity: The gut microbiota plays a crucial role in training and modulating the immune system. A diverse and balanced gut microbiota can help strengthen the immune response, while imbalances or dysbiosis can lead to immune dysfunction and increased susceptibility to infections and autoimmune conditions.

2. Gut Barrier Function: The lining of the gut acts as a barrier,

preventing harmful substances from entering the bloodstream. A healthy gut barrier is essential for optimal immune function. When the gut barrier becomes compromised, as in the case of leaky gut syndrome, it can lead to increased inflammation and immune dysregulation.

3. Gut-Associated Lymphoid Tissue (GALT): The gut is home to a significant portion of the body's immune cells, known as gut-associated lymphoid tissue (GALT). These immune cells help protect against pathogens and maintain immune balance. A healthy gut environment supports the proper functioning of GALT.

Gut Health and Overall Well-being

Beyond mental health and immune function, gut health has been linked to various other aspects of overall well-being. Here are a few examples:

1. Nutrient Absorption: A healthy gut is essential for proper nutrient absorption. When the gut is inflamed or imbalanced, it can impair the absorption of essential vitamins, minerals, and other nutrients, leading to deficiencies and overall compromised well-being.

2. Energy Levels: The gut plays a role in energy production and metabolism. Imbalances in gut health can impact energy levels and contribute to feelings of fatigue and lethargy.

3. Skin Health: The gut-skin axis highlights the connection between gut health and skin conditions such as acne, eczema,

and psoriasis. Imbalances in the gut microbiota and increased inflammation can contribute to skin issues.

4. Sleep Quality: The gut produces various hormones and neurotransmitters that influence sleep patterns. Disruptions in gut health can affect the production and regulation of these sleep-related substances, leading to sleep disturbances and poor sleep quality.

Frequently Asked Questions (FAQ)

1. Q: What is gut health?

A: Gut health refers to the overall well-being of the digestive system, including the balance of gut bacteria, proper digestion, and absorption of nutrients.

2. Q: How does a plant-based diet support gut health?

A: A plant-based diet provides fiber, antioxidants, and a variety of nutrients that promote a healthy gut microbiome and support optimal digestion.

3. Q: Can a plant-based diet help with digestive issues like bloating and gas?

A: Yes, a plant-based diet rich in fiber can help regulate bowel movements and reduce digestive discomfort.

4. Q: Are there specific plant-based foods that are beneficial for gut health?

A: Yes, foods like fruits, vegetables, whole grains, legumes, nuts, and seeds are particularly beneficial for gut health due to their fiber and nutrient content.

5. Q: Can a plant-based diet help with conditions like irritable bowel syndrome (IBS)?

A: Many individuals with IBS find relief by adopting a plant-based diet, as it eliminates common trigger foods and provides gentle fiber for bowel regularity.

6. Q: Does a plant-based diet provide enough protein for gut health?

A: Yes, plant-based sources like legumes, tofu, tempeh, quinoa, and nuts are excellent sources of protein that support gut health.

7. Q: Can a plant-based diet help reduce inflammation in the gut?

A: Yes, plant-based foods are rich in anti-inflammatory compounds that can help reduce gut inflammation and promote healing.

8. Q: Is it necessary to take probiotic supplements on a plant-based diet?

A: While probiotic supplements can be beneficial, a well-rounded plant-based diet with fermented foods like sauerkraut and kimchi can provide natural probiotics.

9. Q: Can a plant-based diet help improve gut motility?

A: Yes, the fiber in plant-based foods adds bulk to the stool, promoting regular bowel movements and improving gut motility.

10. Q: Are there any plant-based foods that can worsen gut health?

A: Some individuals may be sensitive to certain plant-based

foods like beans or cruciferous vegetables, but it varies from person to person.

11. Q: Can a plant-based diet help with leaky gut syndrome?

A: While more research is needed, a plant-based diet's anti-inflammatory properties and nutrient density may support gut healing in cases of leaky gut syndrome.

12. Q: Can a plant-based diet help with acid reflux?

A: Yes, a plant-based diet can reduce symptoms of acid reflux by avoiding trigger foods like fatty meats and incorporating alkaline-rich foods like leafy greens.

13. Q: Can a plant-based diet help with constipation?

A: Yes, the fiber in plant-based foods adds bulk to the stool, promoting regular bowel movements and relieving constipation.

14. Q: Can a plant-based diet help with diarrhea?

A: Yes, a plant-based diet can help regulate bowel movements and provide soothing, easily digestible foods during bouts of diarrhea.

15. Q: Can a plant-based diet help with diverticulitis?

A: A plant-based diet high in fiber can help prevent diverticulitis by promoting regular bowel movements and reducing pressure on the colon.

16. Q: Can a plant-based diet help with Crohn's disease?

A: While individual experiences may vary, many individuals with Crohn's disease find relief by adopting a plant-based diet that avoids trigger foods and focuses on gentle, nourishing options.

17. Q: Can a plant-based diet help with ulcerative colitis?

A: Some individuals with ulcerative colitis find that a plant-based diet reduces symptoms and supports gut healing, but it's important to work with a healthcare professional for personalized guidance.

18. Q: Can a plant-based diet help with gallbladder issues?

A: A plant-based diet low in saturated fats can help reduce the risk of gallbladder issues and promote overall digestive health.

19. Q: Can a plant-based diet help with acid indigestion?

A: Yes, a plant-based diet can reduce symptoms of acid indigestion by avoiding trigger foods and incorporating soothing options like ginger and chamomile tea.

20. Q: Can a plant-based diet help with celiac disease?

A: Yes, a well-planned plant-based diet can be gluten-free and provide all the necessary nutrients for individuals with celiac disease.

21. Q: Can a plant-based diet help with food intolerances?

A: A plant-based diet can eliminate common trigger foods and provide a wide variety of alternatives, making it easier to manage food intolerances.

22. Q: Can a plant-based diet help with weight management?

A: Yes, a plant-based diet can support weight management by providing nutrient-dense, low-calorie foods that promote satiety and healthy weight loss.

23.Q: Can a plant-based diet help with acid reflux?

A: Yes, a plant-based diet can reduce symptoms of acid reflux by avoiding trigger foods like fatty meats and incorporating alkaline-rich foods like leafy greens.

24. Q: Can a plant-based diet help with constipation?

A: Yes, the fiber in plant-based foods adds bulk to the stool, promoting regular bowel movements and relieving constipation.

25. Q: Can a plant-based diet help with diarrhea?

A: Yes, a plant-based diet can help regulate bowel movements and provide soothing, easily digestible foods during bouts of diarrhea.

26. Q: Can a plant-based diet help with diverticulitis?

A: A plant-based diet high in fiber can help prevent diverticulitis by promoting regular bowel movements and reducing pressure on the colon.

27. Q: Can a plant-based diet help with Crohn's disease?

A: While individual experiences may vary, many individuals with Crohn's disease find relief by adopting a plant-based diet that avoids trigger foods and focuses on gentle, nourishing options.

28. Q: Can a plant-based diet help with ulcerative colitis?

A: Some individuals with ulcerative colitis find that a plant-based diet reduces symptoms and supports gut healing, but it's important to work with a healthcare professional for personalized guidance.

29. Q: Can a plant-based diet help with gallbladder issues?
A: A plant-based diet low in saturated fats can help reduce the risk of gallbladder issues and promote overall digestive health.

30. Q: Can a plant-based diet help with acid indigestion?
A: Yes, a plant-based diet can reduce symptoms of acid indigestion by avoiding trigger foods and incorporating soothing options like ginger and chamomile tea.

31. Q: Can a plant-based diet help with celiac disease?
A: Yes, a well-planned plant-based diet can be gluten-free and provide all the necessary nutrients for individuals with celiac disease.

32. Q: Can a plant-based diet help with food intolerances?
A: A plant-based diet can eliminate common trigger foods and provide a wide variety of alternatives, making it easier to manage food intolerances.

33. Q: Can a plant-based diet help with weight management?
A: Yes, a plant-based diet can support weight management by providing nutrient-dense, low-calorie foods that promote satiety and healthy weight loss.

34. Q: Can a plant-based diet help with diabetes management?
A: Yes, a plant-based diet high in fiber and low in processed foods can help regulate blood sugar levels and improve insulin sensitivity.

35. Q: Can a plant-based diet help with heart health?

A: Yes, a plant-based diet low in saturated fats and cholesterol can help reduce the risk of heart disease and improve cardiovascular health.

36. Q: Can a plant-based diet help with high blood pressure?

A: Yes, a plant-based diet rich in fruits, vegetables, and whole grains can help lower blood pressure and reduce the risk of hypertension.

37. Q: Can a plant-based diet help with high cholesterol?

A: Yes, a plant-based diet low in saturated fats and high in fiber can help lower cholesterol levels and improve lipid profiles.

38. Q: Can a plant-based diet help with liver health?

A: Yes, a plant-based diet can support liver health by reducing the intake of processed foods, alcohol, and toxins.

39. Q: Can a plant-based diet help with kidney health?

A: Yes, a plant-based diet that includes adequate hydration and limits excessive protein intake can support kidney health.

40. Q: Can a plant-based diet help with autoimmune diseases?

A: While more research is needed, some individuals with autoimmune diseases find that a plant-based diet reduces symptoms and supports overall well-being.

41. Q: Can a plant-based diet help with arthritis?

A: Some individuals with arthritis find that a plant-based diet reduces inflammation and joint pain, improving their quality of life.

42. Q: Can a plant-based diet help with skin health?

A: Yes, a plant-based diet rich in antioxidants and essential nutrients can promote healthy skin and reduce the risk of skin conditions.

43. Q: Can a plant-based diet help with hormonal balance?

A: A plant-based diet that avoids hormone-disrupting foods and includes phytoestrogen-rich options can support hormonal balance.

44. Q: Can a plant-based diet help with menopause symptoms?

A: Some women find that a plant-based diet reduces menopause symptoms like hot flashes and mood swings, although individual experiences may vary.

45. Q: Can a plant-based diet help with fertility?

A: While more research is needed, a plant-based diet that supports overall health and provides essential nutrients may positively impact fertility.

46. Q: Can a plant-based diet help with energy levels?

A: Yes, a plant-based diet rich in whole foods and nutrients

Conclusion

Optimizing gut health through a plant-based diet is a powerful strategy for improving overall well-being. By incorporating a variety of fiber-rich foods, antioxidant-packed fruits and vegetables, and nutrient-dense plant-based sources, we can support a diverse and balanced gut microbiome. This, in turn, promotes better digestion, nutrient absorption, and immune function.

It's important to remember that transitioning to a plant-based diet should be done gradually and with proper planning. Consulting with a healthcare professional or registered dietitian can provide personalized guidance and ensure that all nutrient needs are met.

Additionally, implementing strategies like incorporating fermented foods, staying hydrated, chewing food thoroughly, managing stress, and considering appropriate supplements can further enhance gut health.

By prioritizing gut health and adopting a plant-based approach, we can experience the numerous benefits that come with a thriving digestive system. Improved energy levels, mental well-being, stress management, and even longevity are just some of the potential outcomes.

So, why not take a step towards optimizing your gut health today? Embrace the power of plants and nourish your body from the inside out. Your gut will thank you, and you'll reap the rewards of a healthier, happier life.

Remember, this book is just a starting point. Continuously educate yourself, stay curious, and explore the vast world of plant-based nutrition. Your journey towards optimal gut health is an ongoing process, and with each step, you'll be one step closer to a vibrant and thriving gut.

Now, go forth and nourish your gut with the abundance of plant-based goodness that nature has to offer. Your body, mind, and overall well-being will thank you for it.

Do this for me

Thank you, dear reader, for taking the time to delve into the world of optimizing gut health with a plant-based diet. I hope that this book has provided you with valuable insights and information to support your journey towards a healthier gut.

If you found this book helpful and enjoyed reading it, I kindly ask you to consider leaving a review or rating. Your feedback is incredibly valuable and will help others discover the benefits of a plant-based approach to gut health.

Furthermore, if you know someone who might benefit from this information, I encourage you to share it with them. Together, we can spread the knowledge and empower more individuals to prioritize their gut health and embrace the nourishing power of plants.

Thank you once again for your time and trust. May your gut thrive, and may you continue to prioritize your well-being through the wonders of a plant-based lifestyle.